Stroke of Hope:

Creating the program you need

to discover the results you want

By Heather Branscombe, PT

Stroke of Hope:

Creating the program you need to discover the results you want

An Abilities Neurological Rehabilitation publication

Contact: therapists@abilitiesrehabilitation.com
Twitter: @abilitiesrehab
Facebook:/AbilitiesNeurologicalRehabilitation
Web: abilitiesrehabilitation.com

The material in this book is intended for educational purposes only. No expressed implied guarantee as to the effects of the use of the recommendations can be given nor liability taken. This book does not guarantee any results. Please consult medical experts.

To Graham, Aaron, Logan and Summer.

You mean everything to me.

Contents

Introduction

Why this book?

I feel like this book is a small way to give back for all I have gained both in my therapy career as well as my life overall. Nothing has inspired me more than working with children and adults with neurological challenges. Working with this population inspires me and has enabled me to learn so much.

We all have challenges. Working with a group of people who often have obvious challenges (but not always) inspires me to create my best life. How can I not participate in regular exercise when I talk about the benefits every day to the clients I see? How can I not set goals and work to achieve them (even when I can't see how I am going to get there) when I see others embracing that very challenge?

While it's true not every person with a neurological challenge has the internal and external resources to overcome their challenges with such gusto, I am awed by the ones that do just that and I want to offer hope to those who are not there yet. There is hope, and the options and opportunities to create better lives after having a stroke are getting better, more efficient, and more effective.

My intention is to write this book as a 'thank you' to those who have helped me acquire the knowledge I have and to inspire further discussion. This isn't so much a 'how to' book as a guide or a framework to help you to achieve your goals.

I recently came across an advance in rehabilitation that was described as a way to "democratize rehabilitation." That phrase really resonated with me. I believe it did so because it resonates with my own core values, as well as the core values of the clinic I founded, Abilities Neurological Rehabilitation.

To have a democracy is to allow people to have an equal say. One of the core values of Abilities Neurological Rehabilitation is to value and respect people. I passionately believe in the right and ability of people with neurological challenges to have an equal say in their own rehabilitation, and therapy programs in general. Only when we become active participants in our care does the care improve and become meaningful. True democracy requires education, and I believe it is my role to educate people and the families of people who have had a stroke to become active participants in their recovery. Democracy is about equality.

Another value of Abilities is client-directed care. What that means is that we believe our client defines what meaningful recovery is to them and we use that guidepost to design a program that meets their needs. Gone are the days of the traditional "medical model" where the doctor was the gatekeeper of all knowledge. The internet has proven a great equalizer and has helped to democratize the spread of information. We as medical professionals can no longer be the keepers of all knowledge. Knowledge and access to it is just getting too big too fast to do that.

Democracy is also about human empowerment. Our third company value is to find a better way. As a physiotherapist, I have a fundamental belief in the ability of people to be empowered physically. The democratization of rehabilitation is simply a way for the very people who are using the program to make the program the best it can be.

In my own practice as a physical therapist, I see myself less as a teacher and more of a coach. The knowledge about stroke rehabilitation is growing at such an exponential rate that no one can know it all. Beware of those who say they can! I feel my best value as a rehabilitation professional is to create the framework for effective rehabilitation and then work with the team (including the stroke survivor and their family) to create the best possible outcome.

Again, my hope is that you can take this framework and run with it!

One thing you need to know about me as a person is that I am a natural big-picture thinker. That makes me different from a lot of physiotherapists whose natural strengths often lie in their ability to pick out the details. I have come to learn, however, that big-picture thinking allows me to make easy analogies that make the education I am delivering easier to understand.

So - in this book I am going to teach you how to create your own physical rehabilitation program by using an analogy. The analogy we are going to work with is that creating an effective physical rehabilitation program is like making a stew. This is no ordinary stew though. This is your own personal stew. No set recipes here! I will help you with the main ingredients but you will decide how the final stew will taste.

As we go through the steps to make your own stew, know that it won't be easy. You will most likely not get it right the first time, or even the second time. However, I know that as you continue to work with this framework and improve the components to meet your own needs, you will be more satisfied and more likely to get the results you want.

How to read or use this book

You may need to read this book twice, if not more, to get the most out of it.

First, I would encourage you to read the book to get and overall feel for it and to get a sense of how all the pieces fit into the whole. You may even be thinking about how this applies to you in that first read, and while I hope you do, I would resist trying to put the pieces together right away.

Once you have read the book and have an overall feel, the second read through will help you get down to the business of the application. My hope is that the second reading will create a deeper understanding and you will be more likely to have a great "first run" at creating your own rehabilitation plan.

If you have a team of medical professionals that are currently working with you - share this book with them! Working together is much better than working in isolation. I guarantee it will be better if you are all trying to head in the same direction.

1

There is HOPE

The number one thing I want you to know, above all, is that there is hope. If you have hope, you have a place to go. If you don't, it's over before it's even begun. When I started Abilities Neurological Rehabilitation in 2007, I had many clients who came to me and said, "My doctor tells me what I recover six months (or a year, or two years) after a stroke is what I'm going to get."

I could see the desperation in their eyes. It was as if they were told there is a fixed period sprint ahead of them and after that arbitrary time, there was no hope, nothing left. It was almost like a death sentence, meaning the death of all future hope of regaining abilities after X period of time.

In some ways, if this were true, it would be better. You could dump all your time, money and energy into that period of X and know that you had done all you could. And it is often true that some people do find that they do recover more abilities in the initial stages after a stroke.

However, stroke recovery isn't a sprint. It's much more like a marathon. While it is true that there may be more relatively dramatic gains initially versus the long term, the current wisdom, backed by evidence, is that there is no end to the possibility of further recovery after a stroke.

Did you hear that?

THERE IS NO END TO THE POSSIBILITY OF FURTHER RECOVERY AFTER A STROKE.

When you think about it, the implications of this fact are much like the implications of running a marathon. How many people run a 5k race for fun but would not run a marathon? Most of us tend to like shorter races because they take little to no time to prepare to just make it through. No one just shows up to a marathon.

On a side note, completing a marathon has been on my bucket list of dreams since I was a university student. It is a huge deal for me. Although I like running, I'm not especially good at it. I don't have that typical runner's body. I'm tall and curvy and built more to tackle than to run. I've always been a middle-to-end of the pack runner and I'm okay with that.

Despite all these obstacles, in 2012 I finally turned the dream of completing a marathon into a goal that was meaningful enough to accomplish. It involved six months of consistent training and there were times when I questioned my sanity. That marathon literally took all I had that day.

The marathon itself involved many more hills than I had anticipated (funny that I didn't anticipate that about a race in Seattle, huh?) and I ended up walking much of the last five to six miles with my husband - in the wind and driving rain. However, I finished, and I even started to train for another one in 2013 - with more knowledge and a better understanding of what I was getting myself into.

I only share that story to show that I have felt a bit of your pain. I know how hard it is to accomplish a goal that seems impossible. And for those who don't think that's a close enough example, I have a personal journey around stroke rehabilitation as well.

One of my three lovely and amazing children had a stroke before he was born. I share that to tell you I am on that marathon in a different way as well. He inspires me, frustrates me, and fills me with a love I didn't even know I had before. Professionally and personally, I have a bit of an insight into what you may be going through. I use this stroke stew as a framework for him as well. More than any other client I have seen and advised, I have gained the most from living with and learning from him. Therapists come and go but family is forever. My hope and intention is to help families to use this framework to increase their own capacity.

But here you are; living or caring about someone who has figuratively "shown up" to a marathon of physical recovery after a stroke without even wanting it. This marathon is going to take a lot longer than five or six hours. It may even take longer than five or six years. There are going to be a lot of metaphorical hills, wind, and rain along your way.

If you are reading this and you are the one that has had a stroke, I would encourage you to use family or friends to help you on your way. Giving them this book to read will help them to understand where you're coming from and where you're intending to go.

If you are the friend or family member of someone who has had a stroke, I would encourage you to enlist help along your way too.

The marathon of stroke recovery

Along your journey, you will have help along the way, especially if you ask for it. It isn't necessary or even better to run the whole way. Walking and rest breaks are fine, and for some may even help them to go farther along the path to recovery.

One of the things I like best about participating in real marathons is that they feed you on the way! For your own marathon of stroke recovery, you will need to know what kinds of "food" fuels you best. As you continue your journey, you will use trials and testing to figure this out.

The purpose of this book is to help you to figure out the right recipe for your own recovery. You are going to learn about an evidence-based framework to create your own recipe. You are going to learn about what each ingredient category means within the framework, and how each category works together.

As new treatment approaches develop, you are going to learn how to evaluate those approaches and how to be selective about which ones you implement into your own program. You will learn how to use other chefs (your medical team) to enhance your program - how to work with them, how to get the most out of them, and when to use them. You will finally learn how to evaluate and revise your program for years to come, so that the possibilities for recovery become what they should be - endless.

So let's get started!

2

Rehabilitation and Creating a Stew -The Analogy

The overall framework we are going to use is what I like to refer to as a top-down approach. This allows a person to use it continuously to get the results that are most meaningful in the context of their own situation.

Remembering that physical rehabilitation after a stroke is like a marathon, we are going to use this recipe as a fuel for our journey. Will the recovery be smooth? No. Will it be guaranteed? Not necessarily. There may be other medical factors that can negatively impact one's physical recovery. However, this is a framework that I use personally and professionally and it is one that others have used successfully to create the desired results.

We are going to assume that if you are using this framework, you are already medically stable. What I mean by that is relatively healthy other than having had a stroke. If you are having medical issues such as uncontrolled seizures, heart or circulation issues such as high blood pressure and/or uncontrolled blood pressure, any broken bones or other medical issues that are under the immediate supervision of a medical professional, please consult that professional before you work with this framework.

I am also assuming that you have a basic understanding about your stroke, how it happened and what it means. If you don't, I would strongly suggest you talk to someone on your medical team as well as use the many resources available about strokes in general to give you a good background knowledge base.

Our framework isn't as much about what happened in the past (i.e. the stroke) but what we are going to do about it (i.e. the physical rehabilitation plan). The framework will be your own recipe to make a delicious, individualized stew. This stew is going to fuel the marathon of recovery for an indefinite period of time.

Each recipe will be unique because each person is unique and will therefore define recovery uniquely to their own circumstances.

The ingredients of this stew will be the basic principles and components of a top-down approach to physical rehabilitation.

It will be delicious because the flavor will be self-selected. This will make it meaningful and be designed to positively impact your life and the lives of those around you.

But wait; let's answer the number one question first...

Is the stew going to be expensive?

There is a perception that money will help buy recovery after stroke. I will be the first to admit I have seen how financial resources play both a positive and negative influence in recovery. This is true in every country in this world and goes beyond political policies about the funding of healthcare. While those political thoughts are way outside the scope of this book, I wanted to take a moment to comment on my own thoughts about financial resources and functional recovery after a stroke.

It is my opinion that finances can impact the functional recovery after a stroke but not to the extent that most people think. In this case, I am talking about after a person has become medically stable and the stroke has left an unchanging impact on the brain - meaning the damage has been done; it won't get better but it won't get worse either. In this case, money can help improve recovery but the money needs to be well spent to have the greatest impact.

Let's get back to the recipe for the stew as a plan for physical rehabilitation. If you were to go to the store and chose ingredients to make a stew based *solely* on price, what would happen? If you went exclusively on price alone, you could end up with an expensive mix that may omit some of the basic items that a good stew requires (no vegetables? no source of protein?). Even if you buy the most expensive item using each piece of the framework, it may not mix well if you were looking at price alone.

Alternatively, what happens if you use some good basic ingredients and then use one or two great quality ingredients for added flavor and punch? The results could be spectacular.

The same holds true for a good physical rehabilitation program. First, above all, we need to ensure you have all the basic ingredients. Next, there may be a way to enhance the program using well-selected quality ingredients that could take your recovery to the next level.

The idea is to not let any therapy approach or flashy tool lead the physical recovery. One should always go back to the basics, which are - what is my goal, and how will this expensive piece help get me to my goal? By looking at expense in the context of the entire program, a better decision can be made about how to use whatever resources are available to their highest and best use.

3

The plan

Choose your base - Setting appropriate goals

When I see people in my office, they often have very vague goals about what they want to accomplish.

On one hand, this is very understandable. When you have had such an abrupt change in your ability to function, anything that you get back feels like a step in the right direction. Or perhaps you have interpreted one of the many health care professional's well-intentioned yet negative messages as a lack of hope.

Some health professionals will set the bar very low. They may not be as current with the latest research or may want to set "appropriate expectations" because they themselves have limited time to work with you.

I am making the assumption, by way of reading this book, your bar is set much higher than that. In my opinion, so it should.

So the first step in creating our stew will be to choose the base of the stew; that is, how to set an appropriate goal that will set the tone for the entire rehabilitation program.

Goals can be tricky things, and even if you are used to setting and achieving them in the past, doing so after having a stroke may seem to be a daunting task. First, take comfort in the fact that setting goals is difficult. It isn't an exact science. You are going to get it wrong. But so do trained medical professionals - all the time. We both underestimate and overestimate goals. In fact, the topic of goal selection is one of the consistent issues I coach and mentor new graduate physical therapists.

It matters less what the goal actually is and more about the intention you set to work towards something concrete. The more concrete the goal is - the easier it will be to figure out if you are getting closer to it or not. Over time I guarantee you will get a better feel about how to set a good goal.

You may have had a lot of experience in setting goals before your stroke. If so, that is great! I would still encourage you to read this section to look at goal setting within the context of stroke rehabilitation. If you have never set a goal in your life, no problem, it is never too late to learn how to do it. This section will show you how to start and I promise you that it will become more natural over time.

What constitutes a great goal?

Most great goals are SMART goals. These goals are specific, measurable, attainable, realistic and with a timetable.

Specific

Think about one or two things that will make your life, or that of your caregivers, easier. What kinds of things can you not do now, that if you could, would be meaningful to you?

Also you may want to think about things that are fun. What kinds of things did you do for fun before? Are there any physical limitations to those things now? What kinds of physical things could you re-learn to do that would make your life more fun?

Specific goals are going to be most effective if they are meaningful and fun to the person carrying them out. The evidence bears that out. This recovery may be a marathon but it doesn't mean you can't have joy along the way.

Some examples of specific goals could be - I want to be able to stand to put my pants on, or I want to be able to run again. This can be the fun part where you can dream so don't rush into making a choice!

Measurable

The next important part is to put some kind of numbers or measurement around the goal. If nothing else, this tells you how close or far you are to reaching your goals.

Again, this can be a tricky part, so I don't want you to spend too much time on this part. We use a measuring stick for the growth of our children but unless there are major issues, we don't tend to get too caught up in the details of how much they've grown over a certain period of time. The measuring stick just gives us something to discuss our results around.

One way to make your goals measurable is to think about the physical goal you have and what you need to achieve that goal. For example, in my example of wanting to stand to put my pants on, I could estimate that it will take about a minute to put my pants on. Therefore, I want to build my standing ability.

If my goal is wanting to run, I may want to be able to run in a 1km race with my family because I used to do that before my stroke and that gave me a lot of pleasure. Or, I just want to be able to run across the street to beat the crosswalk near my home because I know it's a long light and I don't want to have to constantly wait.

Hopefully you can see how adding the measurement component to the goal can start to give life to what you want to accomplish.

Attainable

This is probably one of the hardest parts of goal setting. It will be difficult to see what an attainable goal is for you, and the tendency is to set goals that are a bit more attainable, which may mean setting the bar lower than you should.

In the priorities of setting a goal, while this is important to consider, I would not spend a lot of time trying to decide if it is attainable.

We have no real idea of what the possibility of recovery is after a stroke. With new advances in medical care and therapy techniques, those "attainable" boundaries are going to change every day. It is my philosophy when working with stroke survivors that if we haven't got to our goal yet, it isn't because the person has reached their potential after a stroke. It is more likely because I haven't figured out the right combination of treatment approaches to get the results we want.

Now, this may seem noble, but I don't want to ignore the personal responsibility component of goal setting. I also believe that it really is true - there is no free lunch. In the case of physical recovery after a stroke, we know that the possibility for recovery is there; that is the great news. The less exciting news is that it takes many more repetitions to learn a motor skill after a stroke than it does prior to a stroke.

There are also the individual differences that each person has when learning motor skills that will influence how much they have to practice.

For example, if you put three people side by side in front of a piano and ask them to practice the same thing for the same amount of time every day, eventually some differences will appear. Those differences in how well they play can be accounted for by each person's natural ability to learn a motor skill.

You can see the same phenomenon in athletics. There are many natural athletes that not only take their fitness level from one sport to another, but also take their ability to pick up motor skills quickly from sport to sport.

Getting back to what a realistic goal looks like, we have no idea how many repetitions of practice it will take any one person after a stroke to learn a task, other than it will be a lot. Therefore, your ability and/or willingness to practice and get as many repetitions as you can, every single day, will be a major factor as to how realistic a goal is.

If you have less time, ability, or opportunity to practice, there is no judgment; just know that change will take longer. The more time, ability, or opportunity to practice will lead to more results, faster.

If we go back to my goal of wanting to stand so I can put my pants on, I may only have the opportunity to put my pants on once or twice a day, but I can start to think about my environment and how many opportunities I can have or I can take to practice standing throughout the day. If the answer is very few, then I know that it will take me longer, even though I may still want to pursue that goal.

If I want to run in a 1k race and I have access to daily therapy, a treadmill that I am safe to use on my own, and the time to practice on a daily basis, I know that my results may come more quickly.

At the end of the day, go with what is specific and relatable to you and we will figure out what is attainable, or how to make that goal attainable, as we go.

Relatable

This is where the rubber hits the road. It is the most important part of the goal because if the achievement has no meaning in your life, then why pursue it?

Make sure that the goal is what you want to achieve and not a goal that you think you should be doing. Consider what will make your life easier, more fun, or more fulfilling? How do physical skills play into those ideas?

The specificity of the goal is really the "what" of the goal, while the relatability is the "why." Make sure you have that 'why' firmly in place before you start because that is what will sustain you as you put the time in to achieve your goal.

This may be a good time to talk about visualization. There is very good evidence that visualizing an activity is very similar to the brain to actually physically practicing the event. There is a reason professional and elite level athletes incorporate this into their routine.

It may feel foreign at first, but know that visualization is a skill and like any other skill, you get better with practice. To help add life to your vision, think about the setting you may be doing your goal skill in. What kinds of things or people can you see around you? What time of day is it, how warm or cold is it? What other noises do you hear and what can you touch? Are there any smells that you would expect to have while performing this skill? How will you feel inside as you perform this skill?

As you visualize the setting using all of your senses, it will add life to your visualization and give your brain more input. Think of yourself as a high level performer and you are more likely to fulfill those expectations.

Timeliness

The final aspect of a goal to consider is to put a timeline on your goal. Again, focusing on the timeline isn't super important but it does help us to acknowledge how realistic and even effective our goal has been.

This is as simple as putting a date to the goal. For my standing example, my final goal can read, I want to be able to stand for one minute to put my pants on in two months' time. Or, I want to run and finish the 1k race with my family in six months' time.

If you don't hit your goal by the time frame, just re-evaluate and adjust as necessary. Would I be a failure if it took me three months to stand to put my pants on instead of two months? Of course not. If I didn't finish the 1k race, is my physical recovery after a stroke a complete waste a time? No again. Timeliness helps us to focus our efforts for a brief period of time and to take a massive undertaking such as stroke recovery and put it into manageable chunks.

Short-term versus long-term goals

The only difference between a short and long-term goal is the time it takes to accomplish that goal. It can also be very personal, meaning that one person's short-term goal can be another person's long-term goal. I have no strong feelings about whether or not you set smaller, short-term goals that lead to your longer term goal or not. My main concern is that you find the goal motivating and focused enough so that you feel like you are making progress, however small that progress may be.

You may have a goal that will require you to learn a lot of physical skills that you may not be able to do. In that case, setting some short-term goals about each component will help you feel you are making progress.

Alternatively, you may just want to focus on one month or one week at a time. That is okay as well! Use the timeliness component of your goal along with the measurement part to see how close you are, and set new goals as appropriate.

How many goals?

Be careful about the number of goals that you set. In my experience we can only focus on a couple (three at a maximum) of goals at one time. Too many goals and you end up diluting your time to each goal, which can result in less progress. You may also have goals that don't relate specifically to physical rehabilitation. In this case, less is more. Start with one goal and see how it fits into your life.

Next Steps

Once you have a goal, or at most a couple of goals, we are going to use that base to help choose the rest of the ingredients. This goal is our touchstone around which everything else revolves. If the rest of the ingredients don't complement the base, then the result will be a stew that lacks the right flavor or gives the right results.

For example, if you decide on a beef stew when really a vegetarian stew would be more to your liking, the results of this process are not going to be as meaningful to you. Stephen Covey, in his book *The 7 Habits of Highly Effective People*, refers to this phenomenon as "climbing the ladder only to see that you put it against the wrong wall." Choose the right base, and the right wall, and even if you don't fully achieve your goal, you will be much happier with the results.

Do this now:

What is the one thing, if you were able to accomplish it, would have the greatest impact on your life?

Discuss this potential goal with someone else.

4

Choosing your source of protein: Keeping all windows of opportunities open

After choosing the base or the flavor of our stew, the next step is to add our sources of protein. After goal setting, this is the most important ingredient of the rehabilitation plan for several reasons. Since we are being specific in our goals and in our subsequent plans, there may be areas that we are missing in terms of looking to improve some of the broken parts or impairments after a stroke. We want to ensure, then, that in focusing on a specific goal that we do no harm by neglecting impairments over time.

Everyone, whether they have had a stroke or not, needs a certain amount of maintenance to keep their body healthy. Our body is a 'use it or lose it' kind of system and therefore we need to keep all the windows of opportunity open to pursue new goals in the future.

For those who have not had a stroke, some of these maintenance issues are keeping joints, muscles and heart/lungs in good working order. Most people keep a base amount of joint movement and muscle strength just by doing everyday activities. We used to be able to keep our lungs and heart healthy in the same way as well but due to advances in technology, we now need to create artificial opportunities to keep an improved level of cardiovascular fitness.

After having a stroke, you may need to be more deliberate in keeping the joints and muscles healthy as well. There is also an increasing amount of evidence that maintaining cardiovascular health will help also.

The analogy that I use with clients I work with is that even if researchers did find the magic pill to cure strokes, it wouldn't matter if your joints had been contracted and can't be used, or that you are now so unfit cardiovascularly that you couldn't walk two blocks.

Therefore, before we do anything else to meet our specific goals, we need to ensure that our joints, muscles and cardiovascular health remain as healthy as possible. If you do nothing else because of time, energy, or other constraints, make sure this gets done. It is the number one priority.

Keeping the joints and muscles healthy: High tone versus low tone

When you have had a stroke, you will need to put extra energy into keeping the side of the body that was affected by the stroke healthy. The first thing to consider when protecting joint and muscle health is to look at the tone of the muscles on the affected side(s).

What is muscle tone?

At the most basic level, muscle tone is the number of messages that the central nervous system (essentially our brain and spinal cord) is sending to the muscle to fire. Our muscles don't really work like a light switch with an on and off mechanism. They can be best described as having a dial, like on a gas stove. There is always a certain level of activity that increases in response to the brain's demand for more activity in order to respond to a certain task.

Therefore, muscle tone is a continuum that is affected by the nervous system and can be changed by changes to the nervous system. On one extreme of the continuum, there is low muscle tone. In a muscle that has low tone, the muscle is very flexible and requires a lot more strength (to turn up the flame) to accomplish a given task. It doesn't have enough of the right messages from the nervous system. Many people with Down Syndrome have low muscle tone. They are very flexible (think Cirque du Soleil and putting their legs behind their ears) and often take longer to meet their developmental milestones because they need to be that much stronger to do a certain activity.

On the other extreme of the continuum is a person that has very high muscle tone. If you think of someone with a severe head injury, with arms that are flexed and twisted up to their body, those muscles often have high tone, or too many of the wrong messages coming in from the central nervous system. Some mistake having high muscle tone with being strong, but that is not the case. Strength is the ability to use your muscle in the way you want to perform a given task. When people have high tone in a muscle, it means that the flame is too high, and there is often a decrease in their ability to turn down the activity on their own and to voluntarily use their muscle.

Even in people without a stroke, you can see variations of those with varying types of muscle tone. For example, even though I am athletic, I am genetically predisposed to have low muscle tone. My mom had lower muscle tone, I do, and I can see it in my son as well. What does that look like? Well, if you look at my wet footprint on the pavement, it would look less like a foot and more like an oval blob. I have what most people call flat feet. That comes from the low tone of the muscles of my feet not supporting my arch enough. If you were to look at my preferred standing posture, it would be one where my low back sways and my belly naturally protrudes (a fact that I work on every day!). That is the low tone in my core that doesn't naturally want to support my torso.

On the other hand, I would venture to say that most high level sprinters have a natural tendency for higher muscle tone. When the gun goes off, they are wired and ready to go. They often have higher arched feet and a naturally tighter core (darn those genetics!). They often meet their milestones early (like those crazy children that walking at eight or nine months).

After a stroke a given muscle can have low tone, high tone, or can fluctuate over time. These muscles will then affect what is happening with the movements of the joints around them. By identifying the muscle tone and their influence on those joints, we can keep them as healthy as possible and keep the windows of opportunity open.

Finally, just to confuse you a bit more, some people will confuse the term high tone with spasticity. While high tone and spasticity are often seen together, that isn't always the case. While remembering tone is the natural resting state of the muscle, spasticity is a term that describes what happens to the muscle when you move it. In a muscle with spasticity, the muscle will get tighter if you move it quickly. Move it slowly and it won't get as tight. Tightness that is dependent on the speed of the movement (or what medical professionals call velocity dependent) is called spasticity.

All of these terms come into play as we look at the health of our joints and our muscles.

Maintaining the joints of the hand

Let's take maintaining the overall health of the hand for example. If a person has low tone, the hand will have muscles that are very loose. The main priority is to not overstretch the joints and the ligaments around those joints. This can be best done by positioning and by not overstretching. You don't need to stretch a muscle that has low tone. You need to strengthen the muscle so that it can function in a way that works for you. That may mean training that hand to be a good helper hand, or retraining the hand to be the dominant hand again.

If the hand has muscles that have a high muscle tone, the challenge becomes more complicated. The hand is made up of many joints. If you look at the finger, for example, you can see that each knuckle represents a joint underneath. The high tone of the muscles of the hand means that many joints are affected. Since a muscle with high muscle tone tends to be tight, the obvious solution to keeping that muscle and the surrounding joints healthy is to stretch that muscle. However, how you stretch those muscles will affect the joints as well.

For example, after having a stroke many people with resulting high tone in their hand will stretch their fingers backwards without supporting the palm of the hand. If you put pressure on your fingers only, you can see that the joints where the fingers connect to the hand are stretched more than the other knuckles. What that means is that there is an uneven movement available for one set of finger joints relative to the others. That will make it more difficult for the muscles of the fingers to control the joints effectively.

So what is the solution? Try stretching the muscles of your fingers from a bent position by supporting not only the fingers, but also the palm of your hand. See how all the joints of the fingers are moving by around the same amount? Keeping the relative flexibility of all the knuckles of the fingers intact will have a huge impact on the resulting function of the hand.

As we look at each muscle and identify what kind of tone we have, that will help to guide us on the things that are most important to keep those muscles and the surrounding joints healthy.

Options for keeping muscles with high tone healthy

There are a variety of ways to keep the muscles with high muscle tone healthy. This is not an exhaustive list by any means, and I have no doubt that this list will continue to expand over time. I hope and pray that it does, thereby giving people more options that may be a better fit for their individual situations. What I hope this section does is present some of the options that are out there and set the tone for a discussion with medical professionals on what options may be best for your particular situation.

Stretching and Positioning

The first line of defense is to implement a stretching program for the muscle. Because the muscle will tend to get tight due to the increased messages from the central nervous system, we need to counteract that by keeping the flexibility of the muscle. Keeping the flexibility of the muscle will also help to keep the flexibility of the surrounding joints. If the muscle is tight, the joint will move less. Give the muscle more flexibility, and it opens up more available movement for the nearby joint.

So how do you stretch the muscle? The current available research on how to best stretch a muscle with high tone is to do a low load stretch for a long period of time. What does that mean? When most people stretch at a gym, they are stretching a muscle almost as far as they can for anywhere from 10 seconds up to a minute at a time. Believe me, if you are stretching for a minute, it can feel like forever, especially if it's a really good stretch! This may be repeated a couple to five times, and that is the extent of the stretching.

When you have a muscle with high tone, you need to remember that that muscle is often getting those messages to be tighter from the central nervous system 24 hours a day, seven days a week. If you were to stretch the muscle for a minute, with 5 repetitions, you are now expecting 5 minutes of stretching messages that say to loosen the muscle to counteract 1440 minutes of messages that say to tighten the muscle. If your goal is to get the muscle longer, or even to maintain the muscle length you have, I would say you are fighting a losing battle.

The other thing to consider is that people who have high tone may or may not have associated spasticity in the muscle; therefore, if you stretch the muscle with any speed, the muscle will tighten up and won't be able to get an effective muscle stretch.

A low load stretch then is one that in the moment doesn't even feel like a stretch. How far is far enough to be low load? When a muscle has high tone, there are often two levels of resistance when the muscle is stretched. If you stretch the muscle quickly, spasticity will kick in and we will often call that R1, or the first resistance. That first resistance shouldn't be confused with the end of that muscle's length. If you were to stretch the muscle more slowly, you will most likely be able to get more movement in the joint because the stretch goes farther. That end resistance is often what we call R2. In those with more normal muscle tone, R1 and R2 will be the same. In those with higher muscle tone, there will be a difference between R1 and R2.

Our mission, should we choose to accept it, is to close the gap between R1 and R2. We do that by stretching the muscle at a load which is just at or below R1. Stretch too far and you can activate parts of the muscle called the golgi tendon organ. This is a safety component in our muscle that helps the muscle contract if it is being stretched too quickly. What can be a great safety mechanism in everyday life can be really hard to overcome when it comes to a muscle with high tone. In order to ensure we don't activate that safety mechanism, we are going to do a low load stretch for a longer period of time.

How long is long enough? The research isn't entirely clear, but we know that the longer the better. My impression is at least four hours, up to seven to eight hours at a time. At this point we often don't call it a stretch but we call it positioning. If you think about the effect of lengthening a muscle for 240-480 minutes against 1440 minutes of messages sent to tighten a muscle, versus 1-5 minutes a day, you can see why positioning can be a very effective tool in both maintaining muscle flexibility as well as joint movement.

Positioning

Positioning is something that can be done with a specialized device (such as an ankle foot orthosis or a resting splint) or within the context of your interaction with the environment. One example of this is putting a couple of pillows in between the legs while sleeping to maintain the length of the adductor muscles (the muscles that bring your legs together). Another example is to position the arm on an arm rest when sitting so the shoulder, elbow, wrist and fingers are supported. Finally, another option is night splinting.

In the past I have not been a big supporter of night splinting. We know that sleep is very important for both recovery and motor learning. I would always think about my hamstring muscles, which are chronically tight for me. These are the muscles that, when tight, often make it hard for you to touch your toes. Could you imagine stretching those muscles all night while trying to sleep? Me either, so I was not a great fan of night splinting.

However, if we go back to the idea of a low load stretch for a long period of time, then you aren't going to position the muscle in a position of stretch per se. I often say to my clients, if it feels like a stretch then it is too much! One will never be able to sneak around that golgi tendon

34

organ for that long, and then you will be fighting the stretch reflex - a losing battle for sure, especially when combined with high muscle tone. If you consider positioning the muscle for a low load stretch, then the possibility doesn't seem as daunting. It's more about learning to sleep with a new device, which could be the same thing as learning to sleep with a new pillow - it may take a couple of days, but you should be able to get used to it. If not, I would suspect that the stretch is too aggressive and should be relaxed in favor of just getting used to sleeping with a device first.

Take home message

What I would suggest doing then is to identify those muscles that have high muscle tone and identify ways that you can maintain their flexibility and length by either stretching or positioning. The good news about joints is that they require a lot less maintenance to remain healthy. If they can go through their normal movements as little as once a day, that is enough to keep them free of contractures. If you have tight muscles around that joint, this can be difficult, and that is where a specific program of motions can be used to ensure that the joints go through their normal movements each day, despite the muscles around them.

Other Medical Interventions

Other than stretching and positioning, there are other medical interventions that you may consider specifically to decrease the amount of muscle tone. High muscle tone can be a significant battle in gaining functional physical return after a stroke.

One of these options is to take some drugs that specifically decrease muscle tone. There are many options available, one of them being Baclofen. These drugs can be taken orally or, in some cases, injected directly into the spinal cord. The disadvantage right now is that, besides the potential side effects, the drug is not specific to certain muscles. The drugs will decrease the muscle tone in all muscles in the body, including those that would be considered more normal. Therefore, it can sometimes be tricky for the physician to get the right balance of decreasing tone in the high tone muscles without negatively affecting the other muscles.

Another drug, which can be more specific, is Botox, or Botulism Toxin A. That's right, the same drug that celebrities are using to look younger can be injected into muscles with high tone to temporarily decrease the muscle tone in that specific muscle. The advantage of this approach is the specificity, and the results can be dramatic. The disadvantage, again other than the normal precautions to drug side effects, is that it is temporary and the effects of long-term use of the drug are not very well known. Botox often needs to be re-administered every three to six months, and there is only so much that can be injected into a person at one time. You will need to decide, with your physician, if this is a treatment approach that coincides with your overall rehabilitation plan.

Often these medical interventions are combined with a stretching and positioning program for optimum muscle flexibility.

One final option that isn't always discussed is to use electrical stimulation as a way to control spasticity. This is a relatively new area, and therefore the evidence is not as great, but it does look to have some promise. The idea is using stimulation to either stimulate the opposite muscle group, or even at times the muscles with high tone themselves, to temporarily change the muscle flexibility. This kind of protocol would certainly need to be followed up with a medical professional, but can be a less costly way than drugs to help control the muscle tone.

It is entirely likely that by the time you read this there may be other options. So how do you choose what is right for you? First, I would always start with a basic muscle flexibility and joint range of motion plan. That is just one of those things, like brushing your teeth, that will need to become part of your life.

You may even have a program from when you were first in the hospital or in a therapy program. One of the things I would check is that all the muscles are being addressed. Second I would see if there is any way you can cut the program down in terms of the time you need to be actively working on muscle flexibility. Since we know that there is a very basic and minimum amount that each joint needs to be moved, and most muscles will be kept the most flexible by some kind of positioning program, that means that the amount of time you need to be actively stretching is a lot less than you might expect.

Paring down your program may be something you want to do with a medical professional, but know that we, especially physical therapists, like to be thorough. If we are going to err on a given side, it is often on giving too many exercises. Don't be afraid to ask - what is the minimum I need to do to keep my joints healthy and my muscles flexible?

Options for keeping muscles with low tone healthy

On the other hand, if you have a muscle, or a group of muscles, with low tone, the way that you keep those muscles and the surrounding joints healthy is going to be very different.

Remember that, by definition, muscles with low tone are going to be much more flexible. That means stretching of the muscles is often not required. Knowing that muscle tone does not equal muscle strength means that we know that often those low tone muscles may not have the strength to move the joints through their full range of motion. This means that a joint movement program will often be necessary as well as a program that protects the joints from overstretching.

Joints are often protected from going too far by the muscles that surround them. Their relative flexibility will allow the joint to go through a safe range of motions. When the muscles are too flexible, that level of protection is lost. Joints have tissues surrounding them that are called ligaments. These are tissues that attach two pieces of bone together and are often the last measure of defense against too much movement in a joint. They are made from a stretchy material called collagen and, just like many other stretchy materials, if there is too much tension and they are stretched for too long, they will not go back to their original shape. This can lead to joints that have much more movement than they were designed for, which can result in less function and potential pain.

Where you will often see this after a stroke is around the shoulder. The shoulder joint looks like a ball and socket. It has a series of ligaments that hold it together, as well as a series of muscles that keep the ball in its socket. These muscles as a group are called the rotator cuff and come from around the shoulder blade, over the top of the shoulder to attach to the arm bone.

When the rotator cuff has low muscle tone (another word we use for that is flaccid), it is no longer holding the ball in the shoulder socket. What is most problematic about this is that our arm hangs down from the shoulder. If you don't have the rotator cuff to help hold the shoulder joint into place, gravity is going to continuously pull on the ligaments that are left to keep the joint together. Add this to the fact that all of the blood vessels and nerves that feed the rest of the arm pass by the shoulder, then if the joint does not undergo a healthy amount of movement, (meaning not too much or not too little), there is potential for pain and/or less function in the arm itself.

One way to help the shoulder from having too much movement is positioning the shoulder so that the arm is not hanging from the shoulder joint. When sitting, this can be achieved by supporting the lower part of the arm (without pushing the shoulder up so it's up around a person's ears) with a tray or pillow. When standing, that could mean a sling or some other device to keep the arm from hanging from the shoulder.

On the other hand, having flaccid or low tone rotator cuff muscles means that the muscles are not moving the joint through its full movement. Therefore you will want to move the shoulder joint through a pain-free range of motion. There are many ways to do so, and your therapist may have already shown you how.

One caution I would have is that if you are moving the shoulder through its movements because of the low tone muscles that surround it, you may want to support your shoulder blade as you move your arm. This is because your shoulder blade and your shoulder often move together for the best function of the arm, and if you have low tone in your shoulder, chances are you have low tone around your shoulder blade as well. One easy way to support your shoulder blade is to lie down on your back so that the bed supports your shoulder blade. You can then use your non-affected hand to move your affected arm through a pain-free range of movement exercises.

Now that you have a way to decide what muscles are high tone and what muscles are low tone, as well as a way to keep them, and the surrounding joints, healthy, we should touch on cardiovascular health.

Cardiovascular Health

When we talk about cardiovascular health, we are talking about the ability of your lungs and your heart to be able to support your everyday activities. Even after a stroke or I should say especially after a stroke, keeping your lungs and heart healthy is critical for the endurance you will need for most day to day activities.

Keeping your heart and lungs healthy can be difficult, especially if you have mobility issues after your stroke. However, it can and should still be done. Here are some suggestions to make it easier and part of your program.

First, any program should be cleared by a physician. This is to ensure that you are medically stable and are aware of any medical restrictions we need to consider as you make a plan. Issues around blood pressure, for example, can make it difficult and even potentially dangerous to start any plan on your own.

Second, start slowly and incorporate many consistent but smaller sessions rather than one large session. This will help with the motor skill learning part as well as the daunting part. So for example, you may start with a three-minute walk every day or a three-minute video game that incorporates your arms. Start slowly and with something you can manage on both your good and bad days and then build from that point.

Third, you may either want to incorporate this part of your health into your goal or keep it separate. For example, if my goal is to stand by myself to put my pants on, practicing going from sitting to standing could be part of my way to keep my heart and lungs healthy. Or, I could decide to use an exercise bike that works on getting my legs strong and then practice my goal of standing in different ways later. Consider how much time and/or help you have, the equipment available to you, and what you enjoy when making that decision.

Take home message

If you go no farther than implementing this part of the book, that is fine; actually that is great! You are keeping the windows of opportunity open by keeping your muscles, joints, heart and lungs healthy. Even as a physical therapist, I realize that there may be times in your life when your physical recovery may not be a priority. Other illnesses, family issues, or goals in other areas can put your physical skill development on the back burner for a time.

By implementing these basic strategies, you will be ready to go when and if you are ready to dedicate some time and other resources to reaching a goal around a physical skill.

Remember, this is a marathon, and it's okay to metaphorically slow down and even walk sometimes. Eating this very basic stew now and later you will be ready to add other ingredients for a fuller stew. A base of a goal of maintenance with a protein source of basic ways to keep your options open is all you really need for a long time. It doesn't matter how long the stew simmers before you add the next ingredients, if you add them at all!

When you are ready, the next chapter talks about the next ingredient to add.

Do this now:

Are your muscles on your affected side(s) high tone, low tone, or somewhere in the middle? Take time to list your body parts and identify where the tone is different. If you need help, a physiotherapist or other medical professional should be able to help you.

What are the steps you will take to make sure that your muscles, joints, heart and lungs stay healthy?

5

Add the veggies: Practicing what is missing

Now, no matter how basic but sufficient our stew is up to now, the next parts are the most exciting and will definitely add more joy to your program. A base and protein will get you through, but the vegetables add a texture and richness you wouldn't otherwise get!

So to this point you have set a specific, measurable goal that is (potentially) attainable, and is definitely relatable, with a timeline just so we can measure effectiveness. Your goal is beyond maintenance so now we need to decide how to get you from point A (where you are) to point B (where you need to go).

This is really where therapists such as physical therapists start to earn their keep. I'll let you in on a little secret, though; it isn't nearly as complicated as we sometimes let on. Oh sure, we have the experience of trying various ways from getting people to point B, and we go to courses, conferences, and read journals that help us to know about various options; however, you have an advantage as well.

You know yourself - or you are going to get to know yourself pretty quick! You have experience in knowing how well or not well you learned physical skills in the past. Perhaps you are an athlete and are used to physical activities or maybe you were one of those who was picked last in class, and felt awkward around any kind of sporting equipment. Perhaps you were a whizz at piano; or none of the above. These experiences of learning a physical skill can give you some unique clues as to how you will do best in re-learning some skills after a stroke.

Top Down vs Bottom Up Approach

Before we talk about the how to get you to point B, we should talk a little bit about how medical professionals tend to look at recovery or physical therapy in general.

In general, most medical professionals go to highly-regarded universities and complete a number of educational degrees before they start to work on the general public. When they do start to work with the general public, they are most likely regulated on how they practice by way of their membership in some kind of college (for example, College of Physicians and Surgeons, or the College of Physical Therapists). This is all great, but it can lead to the perception that within a given medical profession (for example, physical therapy), all the professionals would look at a given problem, like how to recover from a stroke, in the same way. We can all recognize that medical professionals may have differences in bedside manner or in techniques, but the common thought would be that given similar personalities and exposure to different approaches, professionals would approach a problem in basically the same way.

That assumption is wrong.

I, for one, think it is a great thing that there are such differences, because different people respond to different approaches differently. What I mean by that is that people come to stroke recovery with a variety of strengths and experiences that can influence any given treatment technique. I firmly believe that a variety of techniques can help a variety of people maximize their recovery. Vive le difference!

It's a bit broad but, in general, most medical professionals tend to look at the problem of maximizing recovery through one of two lenses. This lens or framework will make a big impact on how the medical professional will view a given physical problem and how they will approach alleviating it. It isn't just the difference between a shade, as in between blue or rose-colored glasses, but more likely at what parts the professional looks at first, which parts do they look at longest, and how much importance do they put on the information they see.

The first approach is the bottom-up approach. In this kind of approach, a medical professional will look at the specific changes that have occurred due to the stroke and how to modify those changes to help the overall function of the person who has had a stroke. It is looking at the parts that fit into the whole and fixing the broken parts.

What could those "parts" look like after having a stroke? They could be things like less sensation, less movement in a joint, differences in muscle tone or individual muscle strength. The idea is by fixing the broken parts, much like a car, the person who has had a stroke will be able to function better.

The second approach is the top-down approach. In this approach, the idea of "the whole is more than the sum of its parts" takes shape. It's a more specific approach, meaning that instead of looking at the parts that are impaired after a stroke, they will look at what functions that person with a stroke wants to do and figure out what the gap is between what they can do now and what they need to be able to do to complete a given functional task.

There is a lot more evidence for the second approach, and quite frankly, it makes the road to recovery a lot more fun in my opinion. Keep this in mind, because I am naturally a big picture thinker, my brain works more naturally this way. It also makes it harder, if you are naturally more detail-orientated. The first approach isn't wrong per se, just different.

My main concern in focusing too much on the details is what good is fixing a part if you can't do anything with it? What good is strength in a given muscle if you can't do anything fun or meaningful with it?

To go back to my own personal experience, we are more than the sum of our parts. Take myself for example. I am a relatively normal person with some fitness and athleticism behind me (remember that marathon I completed?). I have at least normal strength and coordination. I have normal sensation and there are no issues with my joints. And yet, if you were to put me on a golf course, I couldn't play golf.

Why?

Well first, because I've had only the littlest of exposure to the sport. I haven't specifically practiced the game, so I am not very good at all. I also don't have a lot of interest in the sport (my apologies to all you golf nuts out there- but it isn't for me!).

So if a professional were to assess me, they may find a lack of specific co-ordination, but fixing my "broken parts" without actually getting me out on the golf course would do little to get me to be a better player. You can work on my coordination until the cows come home, I promise you that alone won't make me a better golfer. If I have no real desire to do well, how well will I actually do? This is looking at my golf problem completely from a "bottom-up" approach.

But maybe my professional takes a different approach this time. Instead of looking more about my "broken parts," this person talks to me about how great golf is and how my life will be better for playing the game well - and convinces me! Then they take me on to the course, and take a look at how I play the game as a whole, giving me suggestions but overall praising my willingness to try. They may give me some specific drills to do, but playing the game is the largest part of my homework. Which approach do you think will result in me playing a better game of golf?

While this example may sound ridiculous because I have no overt brain injury, this is the premise of why a top-down approach is similarly superior in getting results in those who have had a stroke. While we can't ignore the "parts" that have changed after a stroke, the evidence shows us that we will be much more successful if we acknowledge the parts that have changed but focus more on the functional skills that we want to regain.

We have begun to address some of the criteria for selecting our protein in our stew, by keeping the windows of opportunity open.

Now what we are going to do is look at each task and decide what parts are being done and what parts are missing. This will help us lay out the roadmap to get us to that point B. The fancy and technical term we use to define these components is task analysis.

Task analysis

Task analysis may be best described by describing what point A and point B looks like and then running through an example. Again, you may not be very good at this at first. That's okay; I guarantee that with practice, you will get better. This is also another great place to seek help from medical professionals if you have access to them. It is by far my most favorite part of being a physical therapist, because I love the problem solving and creativity that you can use.

The first step is to define, in as much detail as possible, what point B looks like. What are all the muscles and joints doing, and how did they need to move to get there? What kind of strength, endurance, and coordination is required? How much help is being given, and what kind of environment will this skill most often be performed in? What kinds of safety issues are there in this situation? These may be best looked at through an example.

Let's say, for example, I want to be able to stand for one minute so that I can put on my pants. I've decided I have some time to dedicate to this task, because it means that I won't be getting changed lying down, which feels a bit degrading to me even though I understand that many people don't have a choice. I'm going to give myself two months to accomplish this task.

Let's think for a moment what it takes to stand up. Do I want to stand up on my own or with support? Well, I know that eventually I want to stand by myself, but for now I will be happy if I can stand while holding onto something solid. I want to have enough balance to be able to keep myself up with one hand, so that I can use my other hand to put my pants on.

To be able to stand like that, I know I need to be able to put my feet flat on the ground and keep my legs straight enough to hold me up. That means I need to have enough strength to get me to a standing position from sitting and enough balance and endurance to keep me there for a minute once I get to that position. I also need enough leg strength to maybe do a little squat as I put my pants on. I also need to figure out which hand will be holding on and which hand will be putting my pants on, and if I have enough strength to do that (which may be another goal altogether). For the purposes of this example, we will stick to what we need to do with the legs.

So, once we have sketched out at least some of the basics of what you need to do to complete a task, you need to find out where you are relative to point B. This is figuring out where your point A really is. This can be accomplished by actually attempting the task (if you feel it is safe to do so), or by matching the skills identified in point B to what skills you have demonstrated to date.

For example, I may be able to keep my feet on the floor on my own, or I may need an ankle foot orthosis or another device to help me keep my feet on the floor. Once my feet are on the floor, I may be able to pull myself to stand, but I sway to my affected side unless I hold on for dear life. I can't do any squats right now when I am in standing.

Let's identify some of the missing pieces.

It looks like I need more practice getting from sitting to standing, as well as practicing standing without putting all my weight on my stronger side. I also need to practice standing for up to one minute at a time, and finally I need to be able to practice doing little squats while I am standing. Well, that's a lot of practice!

As you can see in the example, you can be very broad in identifying the pieces or very specific. There is less evidence about how specific you need to be and more evidence about just getting practice. Which leads to the next question: how much practice is enough?

The importance of repetition

As has been mentioned before, we know that you can regain skills after a stroke but it typically requires more repetition than someone without a stroke to learn the similar skill. That makes intuitive sense. But how much is enough?

Well, in general we know that more is better, but how you space the practice may be as important as how often.

If we look at more conventional skill development such as learning to read or learning to play the piano, we can look at those principles and incorporate them into skill development after a stroke. Typically those who are learning to read or learning to play piano, practice on an almost daily basis. So yes, daily practice, or almost daily practice, will be important to us as well. I often tell my clients who have had a stroke if you only have 60 minutes to practice a skill in a week (which I hope you would have more time, but for the purposes of this example we will go with it), I would much rather you practice six days a week for ten minutes than for one hour once a week. So spreading out the practice over time is important. But can we spread it out too far? Well, yes we can.

If I were to take my golf example, I could divide 12 hours of practice in many ways. One way would be to practice once a month for an hour; another way would be to practice one hour a day, six days a week, for two weeks. Both ways gives me the same overall practice time but which way will make me a better player?

If I space the practice over consecutive days, I will be able to build on the skills that I learned the day before. If I wait for a month between practices, I will most likely forget some of what I learned last month.

That's where frequent practice, even several times a day, with as many repetitions as possible, will optimize the actual learning of the motor skill.

Fatigue, frustration, or lack of time in a given period can prevent more repetitions than one would want. That is fine; just do more repetitions at other parts in the day. My rule of thumb to manage the frustration level is if you are practicing the skill and you miss the attempt, for whatever reason, three times in a row, then it is time to take a break.

For the brain to learn best, it needs to have a "just right" level of challenge. Too easy and there will be no real learning, too hard and the brain will shut down, contributing to a learned helplessness. Neither is ideal. After three attempts, take a break, and try again later. Coming at the task with a new perspective can help your brain develop new patterns that just may help you get to that next level of development faster.

Another tip I often give is to track your repetitions. You can track the number of repetitions itself or as you get better, the number of repetitions in a set period of time. While the changes will happen with practice, those changes will be slow. It is hard to see progress when you are so invested on a day to day basis. By tracking the numbers, a person can see progress, however small, and be motivated by that progress.

On the other hand, you don't want to be so focused on the progress on a day to day basis that you get frustrated when you don't increase your numbers on a daily basis. The numbers won't increase on a consistent basis, but the trend of the numbers over time should show you the results you are looking for. If they aren't, we should start looking at tweaking the program.

I cannot emphasize enough the role of repetition in a rehabilitation program. In my experience, it is a major factor, perhaps one of the largest factors, in the level of improvement that one receives. Repetition can be assisted in a variety of ways.

One way to increase the level of repetition is the use of assistive devices. This can be a physical device, such as a pole or a walker, or a device that is worn, like electrical stimulation. The main idea is to increase repetition so that the skill can be learned faster. I am therefore a big advocate of those kinds of devices, as well as the way that they can help with a person's level of participation.

This brings us to our next chapter, which is adding the spices to your stew!

Do this Now:

Describe what your point B is. What are the things you need to be able to do to accomplish this task? If you need help, a physical therapist or other medical professional can help you with this step.

Now, what can you do now; meaning describe your current point A. How does this match up to your point B? If you need help, a physical therapist or other medical professional can help you with this step.

How are you going to practice the missing pieces? How can you safely practice them on a regular basis? How can you do this and still do everything else you want to do? Make a list and schedule an appointment with yourself to do it now!

6

Add the spices: Putting the skill back into your life

So far, we have created a pretty respectable program. In our stew, we have a base, protein and vegetables. It is functional albeit a little bit bland. How can we increase our enjoyment? We can do that by adding the spice.

The spice in this rehabilitation program is finding ways to incorporate the skill into your life as it stands right now. Your current ability and your ability to accomplish the desired skill may be a long way off. However, this can help motivate you to get to the next level of development.

This is where we need to talk about another variation of approaches in skill acquisition. We need to talk about motor relearning versus substitution.

Motor re-learning versus compensation: what are you doing and why?

When we think about putting a skill back into your life, we can do it in two general ways. In the motor-relearning approach, we are actually trying to get the person to re-learn the skill. This approach takes longer, it's the marathon, but the result is that the person who learns the skill is independent in performing the skill. That is what makes it worth it.

The other, more quick-fix approach is the substitution approach. In this approach, a device or other method is used to substitute for the movement. For example, some people will have a difficult time bending their ankle in such a way that they can lift their toes up after having a stroke. We call that movement dorsiflexion. The ability to dorsiflex the foot is highly correlated to the ability to walk independently. One way to help a foot to lift is by using an ankle foot orthosis. This is a plastic brace that goes under the foot and extends up the back of the leg. The great thing about the ankle foot orthosis is that it can help to lift the foot for you. However, the disadvantage of this same device is that it's *the device* that is lifting the foot. Since the body is a use it or lose it process, it will generally not work to lift its own foot when a device is doing a perfectly good job.

That isn't to say that substitution isn't always a bad thing. There are times for safety, convenience, participation or other purposes that the choice of a device is completely justified. The key is to actively make that choice and be able and ready to accept the consequences of that decision.

There are increasing pressures on the healthcare system. No matter what country you live in, medical professionals are consistently asked to do more with less. The result of that pressure is that rehabilitation professionals often need to make hard choices. If a patient they are seeing is not making progress fast enough, or they are otherwise limited in the amount of time they have to work with an individual, their approach towards therapy may be altered.

As caring professionals and in the face of limited time, a therapist will ensure that above all else a patient is safe to go home or to wherever they will be placed next. That dedication to safety will mean that rehabilitation professionals may tend to use devices and devote time to therapy approaches that are more compensatory than address motor relearning.

As a physical therapist who has worked in those kinds of institutions in the past, I understand where they are coming from. However, if we are looking for increased skill acquisition, we need to minimize those devices and to see them for what they truly are; temporary fixes that don't address the real solution. They can add some real enjoyment into our lives if used in moderation - just like spices.

The three general categories I would place this kind of approach in would be for safety, convenience or participation reasons. Let's look at these reasons individually to get a better feel for how we can use them.

From a safety perspective, we may want to protect the health of the shoulder joint, because the muscles around it are low tone and can't help, at this point in recovery, keep the ball in its socket. This is where a sling may be helpful to protect the joint until the shoulder muscles become stronger.

Another example may be to have an ankle foot orthosis for walking, especially at night to get to the bathroom.

From a convenience perspective, there may be times that a wheelchair is more convenient to get into and out of a store than walking. Walking may be a goal, but the speed may be a limiting factor. Life is not always conducive to make every event a "therapy event." In those cases, it makes sense to use an approach that just gets the job done.

There are other times where participation, not skill development, is the goal. This is often in social situations. Getting back to the example where walking may be my goal, but if I want to go to Disneyland with my family, my goal of that day may be just to spend time with my family. A wheelchair may be just the spice I need to concentrate on family time and get to the rides faster.

Life is here to enjoy, and the point of this kind of program overall is to give you increased abilities to increase your quality of life. It isn't to subject you to an entire life of all day, every day therapy sessions. By using this kind of approach sparingly, you will enhance your program and increase your enjoyment.

Principles of using spices

There are a couple of principles to use when selecting these spices that can help you not become too dependent on their ability to "fix" your stew.

The first principle is just enough support. When you are looking at a device or approach to substitute for movement, use just enough to accomplish your task, but allows you to complete what skills you can in an effective way.

For example, you may choose to have a wheelchair or other walking device for longer distances, but select the device based on what the goal of the activity may be. If you are using a wheelchair in Disneyland to get to the rides faster, you may not need a lot of support at the trunk and therefore you can still be working on strengthening your middle muscles while enjoying your day. However, if you know that supporting your trunk is a difficult task, you may choose to have a chair that has trunk support. It doesn't mean that you always need to use that support.

Second, look for substitution devices or supports that allow the ability for motor learning whenever possible. One example of this concept for the foot is the use of functional electrical stimulation. In functional electrical stimulation (FES), an external device stimulates the nerves when you want you use the corresponding muscles. That muscle contraction gives you what is often called the "orthotic effect." What is great about FES is that it not only stimulates the muscles, it also stimulates the corresponding sensory and motor area of the brain. This helps develop a motor learning effect over time.

One of the main reasons why I am a great cheerleader for FES is that it provides the orthotic effect for increased repetition, but also a motor learning effect long term for new skill acquisition. Not surprisingly, the evidence for this kind of treatment is really strong as well.

Alternatively, mobility aids such as walkers, canes or crutches can be beneficial as well. There are very few people who progress directly to independent walking after stroke. These aids help to increase the number of repetitions via steps and to progress to the next level of participation. You may need a range of walking aids as there will be times when you want to be practicing developing a new level of balance and coordination and other times when you want to be faster and participate in daily activities.

The kinds and types of approaches and devices are ever increasing, and so a discussion of specific devices is outside the scope of this book. But if you go looking for devices for a certain purpose, then the device will be to fit you, and not the other way around.

Do it Now:

How can you incorporate some of these activities back into your life now? Will you need any assistance to help with participation? Will the use of some kinds of devices help you to participate?

If you need help, a physical therapist or other medical professional can help you with this step.

7

Testing and tweaking: how to know if you are on the right track.

So, hopefully by this point, you have some kind of idea of what kind of goal you might have, and some ideas on how to get you to that point. How do you know if you are on the right track? Just like any cooking project, by tasting and tweaking as we go.

In our section on setting goals, we talked about measurements with a timeline. I would recommend waiting at least a month before you make any major changes to your plan, unless there are health or safety concerns. Just like a marathoner who looks at their watch every minute to check their time, you will get less reliable information if you are evaluating your program too frequently.

So how do you know if it's working? When is the stew the right stew?

Check your results. Are you closer to your goal than you were a month ago? Have you progressed as quickly as you wanted to, given how often you were able to practice? Do you have all the tools you need to get to the next step? What are friends, family or medical professionals saying about your progress (while this is not always the best feedback, it does give you another evaluation point)? What does your gut tell you?

If all systems are go, don't mess with a good thing. If you feel like changes are required, go through the process again. Look at your goal, the base - is it SMART? You now have a bit more information to evaluate the goal itself.

Look at your source of protein- are you keeping all the windows of opportunity open, or are you shirking for the more fun parts of the stew? Is there anything you can add or eliminate to keep your muscles, joints, heart and lungs healthy? If you compromise this part, you won't be able to sustain skill development over the long term.

Look at your vegetables - practicing the missing pieces of the desired skill. Do you have all the missing pieces? Have you discovered more or mastered some as you started to practice? Have you completed more repetitions, or can you do more repetitions in a certain space of time?

Look at the spice - have you incorporated this skill back into your life, even if that means temporarily using substitution or other assistive devices? Are you relying on the spice to flavor your entire stew or do you use it sparingly to enhance the flavor?

Asking those kinds of questions will help you to put all the pieces together. Medical professionals, friends and family can all add their own ingredients but only you know what is best for your own recovery, what is missing, and what the next step is for you. The answers truly are inside you!

Some further thoughts about evaluating ingredients

As you begin this journey about achieving recovery after a stroke, you are invariably going to get all kinds of advice. This advice will come from more "respected" people, such as medical professionals, as well as other well-meaning bystanders. This can include friends, families, and even complete strangers!

There is increasing interest in new approaches and new devices, new therapies and new thoughts on how to heal the brain. Some people are very much into the top-down approach, and others feel strongly that the bottom-up approach is the way to go. Some feel substitution is the best approach while others believe any substitution is wrong and can lead to bad habits that are difficult to break.

You will get emails and suggestions everywhere. "You should try this pill!" "I heard that this is a breakthrough for people who have had a stroke!" "My uncle (son, friend, etc.) tried this and it was amazing!" So how do you evaluate if a new device, approach, or technique is right for you?

First, by starting with your goals in mind. Will this have any advantage in helping me to meet a goal that is important to me? If the answer is no, it doesn't matter how great the ingredient is, toss it! Would the nicest, leanest piece of top sirloin help you create a vegetarian stew? NO! Therefore, it is important to evaluate the ingredient based on what you want to create.

Second, you should take some time to find out what kind of evidence there is behind the ingredient. A lack of evidence does not necessarily mean that it is not effective, just that there is no research to back it up. Conversely, an ingredient could have a lot of evidence but may not be a good fit for what you are looking for.

Most people will look for evidence online, and that is a very quick and easy place to find information. Other ways include asking medical professionals. Be careful though on both counts. I have had professionals tell me they don't use a specific technique because it has no evidence, when there have been many peer-reviewed journals and even stroke guidelines that encourage their use! There are times when medical professionals say, "There is no evidence"; when what they really mean is "I don't know what the evidence is and I may not even be really familiar with what you are talking about."

On one hand, you can't fault medical professionals for not being up to date on every single medical advance. Technology, including research, is exploding at an exponential rate. Medical professional get their own "bag of tricks" based on their approach to therapy as well as their experiences in their own professional practice. There is nothing wrong with a professional not knowing everything. In fact, I love it when clients come to me with new techniques, devices, or approaches I haven't heard of. It helps me to keep up to date.

What is concerning is when a professional fails to acknowledge these limitations and/or covers up those limitations by dismissing an otherwise valid ingredient because of their lack of familiarity. This is where developing a trusted team of professionals, while not always possible, is very desirable. At the end of the day, you should always do your own research.

Beware of research that comes directly from a technique's own website. While it may be valid, there are obviously some potential conflicts of interest. There are increasing numbers of websites that offer third party research about research and are offering guidelines to different approaches, complete with an indication of how much evidence backs the recommendation.

I am very proud, as a Canadian, to say that one of the most comprehensive websites is a Canadian one! Stroke Best Practices (www.strokebestpractices.ca) includes guidelines at every stage of stroke rehabilitation, an evidence review of about every technique imaginable, and a database that is reviewed on a periodic basis to incorporate new research and developments. I highly recommend this website as one way to evaluate your ingredients!

Even if an approach or technique has little published evidence, there may still be some value to using it within your program. Evaluate the pros and potential cons of using the technique, including costs, side-effects, and potential benefits. Only you can decide what will work best for you, and with a framework that includes your own evaluate tools for effectiveness, you can discard the ingredient if you are finding little benefit.

When do I call for help?

This program has been set up so that you, hopefully with some advice from some kind of medical professionals, although that might not always happen, can design, set up, evaluate, and recreate your physical rehabilitation program on your own terms.

In the ideal world, your team of medical and rehabilitation professionals have been helping you to do this since the initial onset of the stroke. This would happen by providing education about stokes, types of strokes and how they affect the body, the general progression of rehabilitation, general principles about task analysis and repetition, as well as some clinical feedback on which techniques seem to be most effective in your particular case. As the recovery period increased, the person who had the stroke, along with their family, would increasingly be brought in as an important part of the rehabilitation team. This would help the person and their family to gain competencies in goal setting and creating and progressing physical skill development programs in a way that works for them. Even as the person who had a stroke and their family became more independent, there would be resources that they could call to get advice.

Sadly, this is not a model, no matter where you live, that often occurs. You may be in a situation where you have very little access to medical professionals who have any experience or knowledge in rehabilitation or you may not have a trusted relationship with your team and are choosing to do things on your own because you feel the care would be better. In either case, it would be beneficial to know when you should absolutely get some advice in your rehab plan:

1. Any increase in pain

2. Any unexplained change in muscle tone (either an increase or a decrease)

3. Any shortness of breath or heart issues (eg. racing heart)

4. Any seizure activity

5. Any acute changes in skin (color, rashes, temperature)

6. Any other unexpected changes in medical status

The most likely person you would discuss these changes is a physician, although if you have easy access to physical therapists, in some regions this may be another good first step. The physical therapist can assess you and refer you to further assessment by a physician if required.

Be sure to mention your physical rehabilitation plan during your assessment so that it can be determined if your plan is having any negative implications on your current medical status.

8

Now what?

Now that you have the overall plan, all that is left is to use, evaluate, tweak and repeat. It will feel hard at first but like many things, it will get easier with practice. Don't give up!

I'd like to hear how you make out with your plan. Feel free to contact me about your progress, your challenges or successes at therapists@abilitiesrehabilitation.com; leave me a message on our Facebook page; or send me a tweet. I am happy to support you on your journey.

I wish you every success as you create the life you want.